WAYS TO BECOME MENTALLY STRONG

Tips on how to be resilient in the midst of troubles

TABLE OF CONTENT

Table of Contents

INTRODUCTION

Mental Strength is the limit of a person to manage pressure, pressing factors and difficulties and perform to the most awesome aspect our capacity, regardless of the conditions in which we get ourselves.

Developing mental strength is principal to carrying on with your best life. Similarly as we go to the rec center to assemble our actual muscles, we should likewise build up our emotional well-being using mental devices and strategies.

Ideal mental wellness encourages us to carry on with a daily existence that we love, have important social associations, and positive confidence. It additionally helps in our capacity to face challenges, attempt new things, and adapt to any troublesome circumstances that life may toss at us.

Mental strength includes growing day by day habits that form mental muscle. It likewise includes surrendering negative behavior patterns that keep you down.

To be intellectually sound, we should develop our mental fortitude! Mental strength is something that is created after some time by people who decide to focus on self-improvement. Similar as seeing actual increases from working out and eating better, we should create sound mental propensities, such as rehearsing appreciation, on the off chance that we need to encounter emotional well-being gains.

Moreover, to see actual gains we should likewise surrender undesirable habits, for example, eating worthless nourishment, and for mental additions, surrender unfortunate habits like feeling frustrated about oneself.

We are generally ready to turn out to be intellectually more grounded, the key is to continue rehearsing and practicing your mental muscles — similarly as you would on the off chance that you were attempting to develop actual fortitude!

CHAPTER ONE

<u>Mental Strength and Resilience</u>

Mental Strength talks about the capacity to remain solid notwithstanding difficulty; to maintain your concentration and assurance in spite of the troubles you experience. An intellectually extreme individual considers challenge to be difficulty as a chance and not a danger, and has the certainty and positive way to deal with what comes in their step.

To be intellectually extreme, you should have some level of resilience, yet not all resilient people are fundamentally intellectually intense. In the event that you consider it a representation, flexibility would be the mountain, while mental durability may be one of the methodologies for ascending that mountain.

Resilience encourages you to endure, and mental sturdiness causes you to succeed.

Mental durability starts when you decide to pay heed to what's crossing your thoughts, without distinguishing actually with those musings or sentiments. At that point, finding the assurance to bring out hopeful contemplations about the current circumstance.

<u>Methods for creating mental strength spin around five topics:</u>

1. Thinking emphatically

2. Controlling Attention

3. Controlling Anxiety

4. Setting Goal

5. Imagination

Likewise with developing mental fortitude, creating mental durability requires mindfulness and responsibility. As a rule, intellectually extreme people seem to accomplish more than the intellectually delicate and appreciate a more noteworthy level of happiness.

Significant characteristics of mental durability incorporate the following: Challenge, Control, Responsibility and Self-Confidence. One may have a couple of these characteristics, however having the four characteristics in blend is the way to progress.

CHAPTER TWO

<u>Mental Toughness Traits:</u>

<u>1. Challenge</u>

This is the degree to which you are driven and versatile. To be high on the Challenge scale implies that you are headed to accomplish your own best, and you see difficulties, change, and affliction as promising circumstances instead of dangers; you are probably going to be adaptable and nimble. To be low on the Challenge scale implies that you may consider change to be a danger, and try not to challenge circumstances out of dread of disappointment.

2. Control

This is the degree to which you believe you are in charge of your life, including your feelings and feeling of life reason. The control segment can be viewed as your confidence. To be high on the Control scale intends to feel great in your own particular manner and have a fair of what your identity is.

You're ready to control your feelings — less inclined to uncover your passionate state to other people — and be less occupied by the feelings of others. To be low on the Control scale implies you may feel like occasions happen to you and that you have no control or impact over what occurs.

3. Responsibility

This is the degree of your own concentration and unwavering quality. To be high on the Commitment scale is to have the option to viably set objectives and reliably accomplish them, without getting occupied. A high Commitment level demonstrates that you're acceptable at building up schedules and habits that develop achievement.

To be low on the Commitment scale shows that you may think that it's hard to set and focus on objectives. You may likewise be quickly drawn off-track by others or contending needs.

The Control and Commitment scales address the Resilience part of the Mental Toughness definition. This bodes well in light of the fact that the capacity to skip back from difficulties requires a feeling of realizing that you are in charge of your life and can roll out an improvement. It additionally requires center and the capacity to set up propensities and focuses on that will get you in the groove again to your picked way.

4. Self-Confidence

This is the degree to which you have confidence in your capacity to be gainful and skilled; it is your self-conviction and the conviction that you can impact others. To be high on the Confidence scale is to accept that you will effectively finish errands, and to accept misfortunes while keeping up everyday practice and in any event, reinforcing your purpose. To be low on the Confidence scale implies that you are effortlessly disrupted by difficulties, and don't accept that you are fit or have any impact over others.

Together, the Challenge and Self-Confidence scales address the Confidence part of the Mental Toughness definition. This addresses one's capacity to recognize and take advantage of a lucky break, and to consider circumstances to be free to embrace and investigate. This promises well since, supposing that you are positive about yourself and your capacities and connect effectively with others, you are bound to change over difficulties into fruitful results.

23

CHAPTER THREE

<u>How to Build and Improve Resilience</u>

<u>1. Ability Acquisition</u>

Getting new abilities can have a significant impact in building versatility, as it assists with building up a feeling of authority and competency — the two of which can be used during testing times, just as increment one's confidence and capacity to issue tackle.

Abilities to be acquired will rely upon the person. For instance, some may profit by improving psychological abilities like working memory, which will assist with ordinary working. Others may profit by learning new side interests exercises through competency-based learning.

Securing new abilities inside a gathering setting gives the additional advantage of social help, which likewise develops strength.

2. Objective Setting

The capacity to create objectives, significant strides to accomplish those objectives, and to execute, all assistance to create self-control and mental flexibility. Objectives can be huge or little, identified with actual wellbeing, passionate prosperity, profession, money, other worldliness, or pretty much anything. Objectives that include expertise securing will have a twofold advantage. For instance, figuring out how to swim or figuring out how to play guitar.

3. Controlled Experience

Controlled experience refers to the progressive openness to nervousness inciting circumstances, and is utilized to assist people with defeating their feelings of dread.

Public talking, for instance, is a valuable fundamental ability yet additionally something that brings out dread in numerous individuals. Individuals who fear public talking can set objectives including controlled experience, to create or gain this specific expertise. They can open themselves to a little crowd of a couple of individuals, and dynamically increment their crowd size over the long haul.

CHAPTER FOUR

SYSTEMS FOR BUILDING MENTAL RESILIENCE:

1. Make associations

Resilience can be reinforced through our association with family, companions, and local area. Solid associations with individuals who care about you and will tune in to your issues, offer help during troublesome occasions and can assist us with recovering expectation. Similarly, helping others in their period of scarcity can profit us enormously and encourage our own feeling of versatility.

2. Try not to consider emergencies to be impossible issues

We can't change the outside occasions occurring around us, however we can handle our response to these occasions. Throughout everyday life, there will consistently be difficulties, however it's critical to look past whatever upsetting circumstance you are confronted with, and recollect that conditions will change. Consider the unpretentious manners by which you may as of now begin feeling better as you manage the troublesome circumstance.

3. Acknowledge that change is a way of life

They say that the solitary thing consistent in life is change. Because of troublesome conditions, certain objectives may presently don't be reasonable or achievable. By tolerating what you can't transform, it permits you to zero in on the things that you do have command over.

4. Advance toward your objectives

In spite of the fact that it is imperative to grow long haul, 10,000 foot view objectives, it is crucial for ensure they're sensible. Making little, significant advances makes our objectives feasible, and causes us to consistently run after these objectives, making little successes en route. Attempt to achieve one little advance towards your objective consistently.

5. Make conclusive moves

Rather than avoiding issues and stresses, wishing they would simply disappear, attempt to make a definitive move at whatever point conceivable.

6. Search for promising circumstances for self-discoveries

Some of the time misfortune can bring about extraordinary learnings and self-awareness. Living through a troublesome circumstance can build our fearlessness and ability to be self-aware worth, fortify our connections, and show us an extraordinary arrangement about ourselves. Numerous individuals who have encountered difficulty have likewise detailed an uplifted appreciation forever and extended otherworldliness.

7. Sustain a positive perspective on yourself

Attempting to create trust in yourself can be useful in forestalling troubles, just as building versatility. Having a positive perspective on yourself is critical with regards to critical thinking and confiding in your own senses.

8. Keep things in context

At the point when challenges gain out of power, consistently recollect that things could be more terrible; attempt to try not to dramatically overemphasize things. In developing strength it assists with keeping a drawn out point of view when confronting troublesome or agonizing occasions.

9. Keep a cheerful viewpoint

At the point when we center around what is negative about a circumstance and stay in an unfortunate state, we are less inclined to discover an answer. Attempt to keep a cheerful, idealistic standpoint, and expect a positive result rather than a negative one. Representation can be a useful procedure in this regard.

10. Deal with yourself

Self-care is a fundamental procedure for building resilience and assists with keeping your psyche and body adequately sound to manage troublesome circumstances as they emerge. Dealing with yourself implies focusing on your own necessities and emotions, and participating in exercises that bring you happiness and unwinding. Standard actual exercise is likewise an extraordinary type of self-care.

CHAPTER FIVE

More Plans for Building Resilience

Gaining from your Past

Investigating encounters and wellsprings of individual strength may give understanding with regards to which flexibility building procedures will work for you. The following are a few inquiries that you can pose to yourself about how you've responded to testing circumstances previously. Investigating the responses to these inquiries can assist you with creating future systems.

Think about the following:

- What sorts of occasions have been generally upsetting for me?

- How have those occasions ordinarily influenced me?

- Have I thought that it was useful to consider notable individuals in my day to day existence when I am bothered?

- To whom have I connected for help in working through an awful or unpleasant experience?

- What have I found out about myself and my collaborations with others during troublesome occasions?

- Has it been useful for me to help another person experiencing a comparable encounter?

- Have I had the option to conquered hindrances, and provided that this is true, how?

- What has helped cause me to feel more cheerful about what's to come?

CHAPTER SIX

<u>HOW TO REMAIN FLEXIBLE</u>

A tough mentality is an adaptable outlook. As you experience upsetting conditions and occasions in your day to day existence, it is useful to keep up adaptability and equilibrium in the accompanying manners:

- Let yourself experience forceful feelings, and acknowledge when you may have to set them aside to keep working.

- Step forward and make a move to manage your issues and satisfy the needs of day by day living; yet additionally realize when to venture back and reenergize yourself.

•   Spend time with friends and family who offer help and consolation; support yourself.

•   Rely on others, yet in addition realize when to depend on yourself.

CHAPTER SEVEN

<u>Ways to Improve Mental Stamina</u>

Mental Stamina is the attribute that empowers us to bear the misfortunes of life. It is fundamental for withstanding both long haul difficulties or unanticipated and surprising battles, concerns or injury, and is just evolved by training and reiteration.

Mental stamina entails organization, strength, persistence, and attentiveness.

Everybody can profit from expanded mental stamina, albeit nobody form mental stamina in a short-term.

Simple tips for building mental stamina over a short period:

1. Think Positively

Fearlessness and the confidence in one's capacity to perform and to settle on choices is quite possibly the main qualities of a sound psyche. Preparing yourself to think hopefully and locate the positive in each circumstance will assuredly assist with building mental endurance over the long run.

2. Use Visualization

Perception is a phenomenal instrument for overseeing pressure, overpowering circumstances, and execution tension. Close your eyes and envision a period that you prevailing in a comparable circumstance. This incorporates recollecting the inclination that went with that accomplishment, not simply the visual.

3. Plan for Setbacks

Life definitely doesn't generally go the manner in which we trusted or arranged that it would. It's critical to recapture center after a difficulty, rather than harping on the misfortune. We can't handle the outer occasions that occur around us, however we can handle what we do a short time later. It's a smart thought to have an arrangement set up that will assist you with managing when things don't work out as expected.

4. Oversee Stress

Our capacity to oversee pressure assumes an enormous part in our capacity to fabricate mental endurance. Despite the fact that not all pressure is terrible — positive pressure (fervor) can be a persuading factor — it has similar actual consequences for our bodies.

Valuable strategies for overseeing pressure incorporate contemplation and reformist muscle unwinding. Recall that you are in charge of your psychological state, and how you will deal with the current matter.

5. Get More Sleep

Getting sufficient rest is indispensable to our physical and mental working in regular daily existence. Adequate rest can assist with on-the-spot dynamic and response time. An adequate measure of rest is supposed to be six to eight hours, or more.

47

CHAPTER EIGHT

How to achieve Resilient Relationships

Flexibility is a vital part of any relationship. Connections require continuous consideration and development, particularly during seasons of misfortune. Have you at any point considered what makes a few companionships or sentimental connections bound to make due than others?

Components which appear to encourage strength seeing someone, and improve their probability of endurance.

Important Feature of Highly Resilient Relationships

1. Dynamic Optimism

Dynamic good faith isn't simply trusting that things will end up great, rather, it is accepting that things will end up great and afterward making a move that will prompt a superior result. In a relationship, this implies a consent to stay away from basic, destructive, negative remarks, and to all things considered, cooperate to tackle the force of a positive inevitable outcome.

2. Trustworthiness, Integrity, Accepting Responsibility for One's Actions, and the Willingness to Forgive

At the point when we focus on tolerating duty regarding our activities, being faithful to each other and pardoning one another (and ourselves), we will undoubtedly develop versatility inside our connections. This incorporates the familiar proverb that trustworthiness is the best approach, paying little mind to the result and outcomes.

3. Conclusiveness

This implies daring to make a move, in any event, when the activity is disagreeable or incites nervousness in a relationship. Unequivocal activity now and then methods leaving a poisonous relationship or one that isn't serving you well any longer, customarily advancing one's very own flexibility.

4. Constancy

Industriousness is to persist, particularly notwithstanding demoralization, misfortunes, and disappointments. It is significant seeing someone to recall that there will great occasions just as difficult situations.

5. Restraint

In accordance with connections, the capacity to control driving forces, oppose enticements and postpone delight are unmistakably significant characteristics. Poise causes one to evade rehearses that will adversely affect their relationship, while advancing solid practices, particularly notwithstanding affliction.

6. Genuine Communication

The most troublesome discussions to have are the main ones.

CHAPTER NINE

How to Become Resilient for Life

In the event that you need to get tough forever, it's ideal to begin with building your flexibility right now! Practice and obligation to the techniques and tips examined above, will over the long haul increment your capacity to bob back and adjust whenever life has given you difficulties.

The silver covering to encountering unfavorable life occasions is that the more you can utilize your versatility muscle, the

better you will actually want to bob back.

CHAPTER TEN

<u>Ways to Get a More Confident Mind</u>

Certainty is one of the qualities of mental durability! Supporting a positive self-view and creating trust in your capacity to tackle issues and in heeding your gut feelings, is one of the principle factors in building strength. So how would we develop a more certain brain?

The following are straightforward ways that you can start constructing your certainty:

1. Complete Things

Certainty and achievement go inseparably. Achieving objectives, and in any event, making little strides towards your objectives, can help construct your confidence and trust in your capacities.

2. Screen Your Progress

When pursuing an objective, enormous or little, it is essential to separate it into more modest, more sensible advances. In doing as such, one will think that its simpler to screen their advancement and assemble certainty as they see the improvement occurring progressively. It assists with measuring your objectives, just as the significant strides towards those objectives.

3. Make the best decision

Exceptionally certain individuals keep an eye on live by a worth framework and settle on choices dependent on that esteem framework, in any event, when it's not really to their greatest advantage. At the point when your choices are lined up with your most noteworthy self, it can develop a more sure brain.

4. Exercise

Exercise benefits your actual body as well as your brain also. Mental advantages of activity incorporate improved center, memory maintenance, and stress and nervousness the board. Exercise is additionally said to forestall and help in wretchedness. Certainty from practicing comes from the physical, obvious advantages yet in addition from the psychological advantages.

5. Be Fearless

To be courageous chasing after your fantasies and objectives requires a degree of certainty. On the other hand, testing yourself by making a plunge into things that alarm you, will assist with building your certainty. Regularly when we set large objectives for ourselves it is not difficult to get overpowered and be unfortunate of disappointment. In these occasions, it is essential to get together your fortitude and simply continue onward, slowly and carefully.

6. Support Yourself

To support yourself when somebody discloses to you that you can't achieve something is a viable method to build up your certainty. Really frequently we may wind up accepting the downers, as they are repeating oneself uncertainty we might be hearing in our minds. To sustain a positive self-see is to supplant those negative considerations with positive ones.

7. Complete the task

Finishing on the thing you say you will do, not just assists with acquiring the admiration of others yet in addition regard for and trust in yourself. Building up your finish abilities will likewise assist you with achieving your objectives and likely fortify your connections, as well.

8. Think Long-term

Customarily, we exchange long haul satisfaction for more prompt delight. We can develop our certainty by settling on penances and choices dependent on long haul objectives as opposed to momentary solaces. Finding the control to do so will get more prominent bliss the long haul and a higher probability of accomplishing the objectives you've set for yourself.

9. Try not to Care What Others Think of You

It is not difficult to fall into the snare of considering others' opinion about you, yet recollect that what others think really makes no difference chasing after your fantasies. Assemble your certainty by having faith in yourself and proceeding to push ahead, in any event, when others probably won't concur with you.

10. Put resources into what Makes You Happy

At the point when we set aside effort for self-care and doing the things that bring us euphoria, it assists with advancing our lives and turns into our best selves. Certainty comes when we are lined up with our most elevated selves and glad for it.